HOW TO SAVE MONEY WITH DIY BEAUTY TREATMENTS AT HOME

by She Rise inc.

**FACIAL | SCRUBS | MASKS | MOISTURIZERS | LIGHT
THERAPY**

Table of Contents
INTRODUCTION

INTRODUCTION

You'll want your skin to seem and feel flawless, if you're like me. I feel a decent facial will assist me in accomplishing this by both postponing and repairing the indications of aging, treating acne and general care for your skin. Facials are a great way of doing this. Visiting Spas or purchasing products can get very expensive so I'll walk you through making result producing products in the comfort of your home. But what exactly is a facial?

What are Facials?

Facials are an excellent method to improve your looks while also providing you with some "me" time. A facial is a simple and relaxing technique that usually enhances the appearance of the skin on the face. There are many different kinds of facials and treatments, but you want to choose one that is healthy for your skin. Whether our skin is dry, oily, or a combination of the two, a proper facial will work to balance out the tone and texture of the face when the right products and treatments are used.

A facial is used to eliminate the appearance of facial defects such as wrinkles, scars, and blemishes by removing the outer skin layers. When a facial treatment is finished, you will feel firmer and more supple in your facial skin, as well as a sensation of regeneration and well-being from the stimulation provided by this beauty therapy. Regular facials remove toxins from the skin and maintain it appearing smooth and refreshed.

Although facials are considered cosmetic operations, they are simpler, less expensive, and require less time to complete than most other cosmetic operations. A facial is suitable for almost everyone because it is non-invasive, causes no discomfort, and can be finished in a short period of time.

Although the face is the most frequently treated area with a facial, other parts of the skin such as the neck, hands, back, shoulders, and chest may also be treated. These other skin areas can benefit from treatment because they are frequently exposed to the weather and are prone to blemishes and other facial-specific disorders.

Depending on the type of skin and the anticipated outcomes, many products and procedures may be used in its execution. Cleansers, masks, peels, and moisturizing agents are all common facial products. Steam, blemish extraction, and massage are all possible procedures. Before your facial begins, you must first determine which sort of facial is best for you. The factors that go into establishing the optimal facial for your specific needs include skin type, age, and the treatments you want.

Benefits of Facials

Nowadays, with increased pollution and a hectic lifestyle, our bodies are constantly under stress. The effects of stress and air pollution can be seen on your skin. Skin disorders are quite prevalent. Facials are one of the few methods available to help you cope with these issues. Instead of viewing it solely as a beauty treatment, it is critical to consider the benefits of facials.

Facials have a plethora of benefits that can help maintain your skin clean and healthy. You should get facials often. <u>Here are some of the benefits:</u>

- **Deep Cleansing**

A cleansing facial will assist your skin in removing oil accumulation, pollutants, and debris from your daily environment, as well as fully eradicating all microorganisms that may cause skin disorders. A good exfoliation, such as microdermabrasion, will remove dead skin cells from the surface of your skin and unclog your pores, allowing other products to be absorbed. This will also help your skin look and feel softer and smoother, allowing your makeup to mix more easily and effectively.

Extraction, if necessary, is excellent for removing blackheads, whiteheads, and pimples as well as preventing outbreaks. This is a must-do step for anyone suffering from acne because it clears the skin and has a purifying impact.

- **Anti-Aging**

Facial treatments can help halt the aging process and prevent wrinkles from appearing. Massaging your face with an anti-aging lotion will immediately stimulate blood circulation and oxygen flow, promoting collagen formation and improving skin elasticity. This results in the reduction and prevention of fine lines and wrinkles. Remember, it's never too early to start caring for your skin.

- **Unwinding**

Massages are excellent for unwinding, alleviating tension, and rebalancing the mind. Your face muscles, like your body, require massage, and most facial treatments involve one. The increased circulation will activate lymphatic vessels and purify your skin, making it appear healthy and youthful. The pleasant aroma of face masks is just another wonderful element to a calming, relaxing experience.

- **Rejuvenation of Skin**

During facial treatment, exfoliation, extraction, massage, steam and masking lead to the recovery of the skin or a fresh, renewed complexion. This improves the skin's appearance by providing it a healthy, vibrant shine and a balanced complexion. You may not see immediate improvements, but your skin will be regenerated in the long run. So keep in mind that keeping up with your facials on a regular basis is essential.

- **Skin Care Routine Enhancement**

A good esthetician will examine your skin and assist you in selecting the finest face treatment for your skin type. You may receive some good advice from a specialist, discuss your daily skin care routine, and obtain recommendations on which products would be ideal for your skin. This is significant because you may utilize these strategies to avoid future problems and keep your skin in good condition.

The specialist will diagnose any skin problems and notify you if there are any changes in moles or suspicious spots that could be a symptom of a more serious skin problem that requires the attention of a medical professional.

- **Treating a Wide Range of Skin Issues**

Getting a regular facial treatment after being diagnosed with a skin disease will help treat and repair your skin. With the correct face treatment, issues such as blackheads, whiteheads, pimples, sunspots and sun damage, acne, inflammation and redness, rosacea, dryness, wrinkles, acne scarring, loss of firmness and elasticity can be mitigated or totally cured.

CHAPTER1: AROUND THE HOUSE PRODUCTS

Skin care products have to be among the most perplexing and daunting items in the personal care aisle. Companies sell "systems" that include different (and costly.) lotions for day and night, cleansing and toning, moisturizing and firming. You can spend hundreds of dollars on different products for different times of day, seasons, and regions of your body. And you can spend a great deal of time considering whether these objects are actually as natural as they promise.

Things In The Kitchen

Or you can go into your kitchen and grab something off the shelf or from the fridge that you know doesn't include any chemicals or additives and works just as well as that $50-a-half-ounce product from the shop at making your skin look dewy and glowing. Most of them have various applications as well.

Olive oil

Olive oil, like many of these edible beauty items, is versatile and may be used in a variety of ways. It can be used in place of more expensive "cuticle oil" to soften and smooth your hands. It's a makeup remover and moisturizer in one. It's extremely effective on dry, scaly areas like the elbows, knees, and feet, and it softens the sensitive skin around your eyes just as well as any expensive "eye cream." You may also use it as an all-purpose, leave-on moisturizer on your legs, hands, neck, and face.

Honey

If you need a little additional moisturizing punch in spots that are so dry they're cracking, rub on a thin layer of honey and let it sink in before wiping away the gooey excess. It's a tad sticky, but it's especially good for winter's ravages—chapped lips and cracked feet. It also contains minerals and antioxidants that nurture and radiate the skin. It also mixes well with fruits and vegetables, such as avocado, to form a face mask.

Avocado

You don't have time or money to go to the spa? Make an avocado face mask in your kitchen. Mash it up and combine it with one of the other ingredients specified above, such as honey, olive oil, or egg whites. Its oil penetrates the skin deeply, bringing the vitamins and antioxidants found in the fruit with it. Many people say that it lowers the appearance of aging as well as skin irritations such as acne, rashes, eczema, and sunburn.

Oatmeal

It's beneficial for you, so eat it for breakfast and then use it on your face as a scrub to gently exfoliate dead skin. It's one of several goods on your kitchen shelf that can function as an exfoliant—sugar, ground almonds, and coffee are three others—but it's one of the best due to its moisturizing properties. To lessen the harshness of the others, you should mix them with some form of oil.

Cucumbers

This is undoubtedly something you've heard before, and it's true. If you've had too many late nights and not enough sleep, it will show in the dark circles and puffiness around your eyes. Position a slice of cucumber on each eye and lie down to tighten the skin. Its ascorbic acid will take out the excess moisture that causes your eyes to appear puffy while also nourishing your face. It can also be used to relieve the sting of a sunburn.

Lemon juice

Do you require a skin toner? Don't buy a pricey product that contains fragrance and maybe drying alcohol. Simply apply some lemon juice on your skin for 10 to 15 minutes before rinsing. It will not only tighten your skin, but it will also lighten blemishes, scars, freckles, and other discolored areas. Its antimicrobial and astringent characteristics can aid in the prevention of outbreaks.

Things In The Bathroom

Essential oils

They are manufactured from plant parts such as leaves, herbs, barks, and rinds. Concentrating them into oils is done in a variety of ways. You can incorporate them into vegetable oils, lotions, or bath gels. Alternatively, you may smell them, massage them on your skin, or put them in your bath.

Other Oils

1. **Coconut Oil:** Coconut oil absorbs quickly into the skin and is believed

to offer numerous health advantages, including those from vitamins E and K, as well as antifungal and antibacterial characteristics.

2. **Olive Oil**: Olive oil is not known to cause allergy reactions in most people. However, for the greatest results, use extra-virgin olive oil. Olive oil is abundant in A, D, E and K vitamins and can be employed as a moisturizer. It is an excellent choice for an all-over application due to its thick consistency.

3. **Sunflower Seed Oil**: Sunflower seed oil is readily available, abundant in vitamin E, and easily absorbed into the skin, making it an excellent natural moisturizer.

4. **Shea Butter:** Shea butter is a tallow-like material that is often available in a solid form but melts at body temperature and is occasionally used as a moisturizer and hair product. To achieve a smoother texture for application, unrefined, organic shea butter can be blended with olive oil or coconut oil.

5. **Jojoba Oil:** Among other skin benefits, jojoba oil has anti-inflammatory and wound-healing properties.

6. **Grapeseed Oil:** Grapeseed oil, which contains vitamin E and vital fatty acids, is light in comparison to other natural oils. It also has anti-inflammatory, anti-microbial, and antioxidant effects.

7. **Rose Hip Seed Oil:** This oil's essential fatty acids and antioxidants, including provitamin A, offer moderate protection against inflammation and oxidative skin damage.

Vitamin creams

Skin care should be an important aspect of your overall health regimen. After all, it is your body's largest organ.

The first thing most doctors will encourage you to do to keep your skin healthy is to limit your exposure to the sun's damaging ultraviolet (UV) radiation and to apply protective sunscreen when you are outside.

But the sun isn't without its benefits. Just 10–15 minutes of exposure per day aids in the production of vitamin D throughout the skin. Vitamin D, along with vitamins C, E, and K, is one of the finest vitamins for your skin.

- **Vitamin D**

When sunlight is absorbed by your skin, it produces vitamin D. When this happens, cholesterol turns to vitamin D. Vitamin D is subsequently absorbed by your liver and kidneys and transported throughout your body to aid in the formation of healthy cells. This includes the skin, where vitamin D is essential for skin tone. It may possibly aid in the treatment of psoriasis.

- **Vitamin C**

Vitamin C is abundant in both the epidermis (outer layer of skin) and the dermis (inner layer of skin). Its anti-cancer (antioxidant) capabilities, as well as its involvement in collagen creation, help to keep your skin healthy. As a result, vitamin C is a major element in many anti-aging skin care treatments.

Oral vitamin C supplementation can boost the effectiveness of sunscreens applied to your skin to protect it from the sun's harmful UV rays. It accomplishes this by reducing cell damage and assisting in the repair of body wounds. Because of its critical function in the body's natural collagen synthesis, vitamin C can also help prevent the indications of aging. It aids in the healing of injured skin and, in some situations, the appearance of wrinkles. A sufficient intake of vitamin C can also aid in the repair and prevention of dry skin.

- **Vitamin E**

Vitamin E, like vitamin C, is an antioxidant. Its primary role in skin care is to protect the skin from sun damage. Vitamin E absorbs harmful UV rays of the sun when applied to the skin. The ability of the body to reduce the damage produced by UV rays is referred to as photoprotection. This can aid in the prevention of dark patches and wrinkles.

Vitamin E is normally produced by the body through sebum, an oily material secreted via the pores of the skin. Sebum, in the proper proportion, helps to keep the skin conditioned and avoids dryness. Vitamin E can compensate for a lack of sebum if you have very dry skin. Vitamin E may also be used to reduce inflammation of the skin.

- **Vitamin K**

Vitamin K is necessary for the body's blood clotting mechanism, which aids in the healing of wounds, bruises, and surgical sites. <u>The basic functions of vitamin K are also known to aid in the treatment of some skin disorders, such as:</u>

- ☐ Stretch marks
- ☐ Stubborn circles under your eyes
- ☐ Spider veins
- ☐ Scars
- ☐ Dark spots

Vitamin K can be found in a variety of topical treatments for the skin and can aid in the treatment of a number of skin diseases. Doctors routinely use vitamin K lotions on patients who have just had surgery to assist minimize swelling and bruising. This may assist to accelerate skin healing.

Aloe Vera

When you get a bad sunburn, the first thing that comes to mind is applying Aloe Vera gel on your burned skin. The plant Aloe Vera is well-known for its medical and cosmetic properties. This gooey superhero not only soothes sunburns, but it also aids in the treatment of a variety of skin ailments such as frostbite, psoriasis, cold sores, and more.

When applied to the face, aloe vera can help hydrate the skin. Applying a small bit of aloe vera to the face on a regular basis can help heal a variety of skin disorders, including acne and eczema.

CHAPTER 2: MAKING SCRUBS AND MASKS

Making your own bath and body products at home, such as body scrubs, bath salts, facial masks, and more, is simple and good for your skin. You will not only save a lot of money by making these products at home, but you will also know exactly what is going on your skin. This is significant since roughly 60% of the substances applied to our skin are absorbed into our circulation. The lower the number of substances we expose our bodies to, the healthier. Because of these factors, you should think about taking up this hobby.

Natural skin care is quite important. Chemicals are present in almost everything these days, from the food we consume to the air we breathe. Making your own DIY skin care products is a simple approach to decrease your exposure to them, and it is rather easy to do. You don't need any particular equipment to get started, and in many cases, a bowl and some measuring tools will suffice. The most crucial thing you need are high-quality products and great recipes, both of which are easily accessible.

Aside from the health benefits to your skin, another factor to consider is the amount of money you can save. The majority of the money you pay for retail bath and body items goes to advertising. Companies spend a lot of money promoting these products in order to appeal to our senses. You may get the same materials for a fraction of the price and save nearly 80% off what you would pay in a retail shop.

The final consideration for homemade bath and body products is that they can be given as gifts to friends and family. This is yet another approach to save money while giving a personalized gift from the heart that matches that person's personality. Who knows, it might even turn out to be a second source of money for you. Every woman enjoys some kind of body product, and the industry is massive. Give it a shot.

Facial Sugar Scrub

Although sugar is not good for your insides, a sugar scrub can be quite beneficial to your skin. Those pricey scrubs in department shops and spas...

they're made for pennies. Sugar scrubs are a basic beauty recipe that may be highly hydrating and exfoliating to the skin.

To slough off dead skin and hydrate, I use scrubs on my face, body, and (particularly) feet. What was the end result? With little effort, you can have silky skin.

If you're new to making your own beauty products (or even if you're a seasoned natural beauty alchemist), I highly recommend giving these homemade sugar scrub recipes a try.

Recipe For A Facial Sugar Scrub

This is an excellent recipe for those who are new to beauty DIY. Sugar scrubs are easy to produce and may be customized with a variety of ingredients to achieve the desired result.

Ingredients

- [ ] 1 cup granulated sugar, white or brown, ideally organic
- [ ] ½ cup oil (olive and coconut oil work well)
- [ ] essential oils of your choice (optional)
- [ ] 1 tiny glass mason jar with a wide mouth

Instructions

1. Combine all ingredients in an airtight container, such as a mason jar.
2. In the shower, use 1 tablespoon as needed. Scrub the mixture into your skin and rinse thoroughly. It will leave your

skin feeling as soft as silk. Goodbye dry skin.

Doesn't that sound easy? Yes, it is.

Variations on Sugar Scrub

Are you ready to shake things up? Adapt your sugar scrub to the season. All of these variations make use of simple items that can be obtained at most grocery stores.

- **Pumpkin Pie Scrub:** 1 cup brown sugar, ½ cup coconut oil, ½ teaspoon vitamin E oil, and ½ teaspoon pumpkin pie spice (or just ½ teaspoon cinnamon)

- **Vanilla Brown Sugar Scrub:** 1 cup brown sugar, ½ cup almond oil, ½ teaspoon vitamin E oil, and 1 teaspoon real vanilla essence

- **Lemon Sugar Scrub:** Excellent after-dishwashing hand scrub. ½ cup olive oil, ½ teaspoon vitamin E oil, 15-20 drops (or more) lemon or orange essential oil

- **Gentle Lavender Sugar Scrub for Face:** ½ cup almond oil, ½ teaspoon vitamin E oil, ½ teaspoon real vanilla extract, and 15 drops lavender essential oil.

Benefits Of Sugar Scrub

On Skin

- Aside from pampering you with natural ingredients at an incredibly low cost, a sugar scrub is an excellent alternative for exfoliating and smoothing your skin, even if it is particularly sensitive.

- Sugar scrubs naturally prevent skin aging by brightening tired, dull-looking skin and promoting healthy, smooth, and beautiful skin.

- To assist remove ingrown hairs, use a sugar scrub in a circular motion on your skin, which is less abrasive than a back and forth motion.

- Sugar Scrubs make excellent gifts for family and friends, as well as party favors.

On Face

There are numerous benefits to using sugar scrubs on the face.

It is a natural humectant as well as a fantastic exfoliant, which helps to remove dead skin cells from your face, lips, and even your body to rejuvenate and revitalize weary, congested pores. As a result, it does not deplete skin of moisture and leaves it delightfully hydrated.

Facial Salt Scrub

Salt contains antimicrobial qualities that can aid with a variety of skin issues. Because salt is a natural preservative, the sea salt scrub will be able to last for a long time.

Recipe For A Facial Salt Scrub

Because coarse sea salt can be too abrasive on your skin, use ground sea salt. For delicate skin, sea salt scrubs may be overly harsh. Also, if you have a cut on your skin, use caution because the salt can sting.

Because salt has no aroma, you may want to add some essential oils to your DIY salt scrub:

Ingredients

- [ ] 1/2 cup oil of your choice
- [ ] 1/2 cup sea salt
- [ ] essential oils (optional)

Instructions

1. In a mixing dish, combine sea salt and oil.
2. Thoroughly combine. If necessary, add more salt or oil to achieve the desired consistency.
3. If preferred, add one or two drops of your chosen essential oil to the mixture and whisk it in.
4. Spoon the scrub into a jar after you're happy with the consistency and aroma.

Benefits of a Salt Scrub

We frequently hear about the benefits of exfoliating our faces. Dead skin cells accumulate and can plug pores, causing acne. That is why exfoliating your face a few times a week is recommended. What about our bodies, though? Our bodily skin also accumulates dead skin cells, which many people neglect and never exfoliate. You can exfoliate your skin by various techniques, one with a salt scrub.

A salt scrub is beneficial because it not only exfoliates the skin (resulting in smoother, softer, and healthier skin), but it also promotes detoxification. A salt scrub can enhance our bodies' natural detoxification processes by activating the lymphatic system, allowing us to discharge stagnant poisons in our systems.

Facial Mask

There are three types for three different skin needs:

- Nourishing
- Brightening
- Clarifying

Also included are suggestions for which essential oils to add to each one for best skin health benefits.

Because honey acts as a humectant(aka it helps pull moisture into the skin), I enjoy using it in face masks. Keeping skin hydrated is essential, especially as we age as our skin becomes drier and loses elasticity. Honey cleanses, hydrates, and exfoliates gently, making it an excellent multi-tasking ingredient.

You can keep it simple by following the fundamental recipe below (or simply using honey on its own). But it's also a lot of fun to combine it with other components to make personalized masks that are tailored to your specific skincare needs. As with any mask, I wouldn't apply it every day, but 1-3 times per week works great

Recipe For A Facial Mask

Basic Honey Mask Recipe

Ingredients

- [ ] 2-3 tablespoons honey

Instructions

- [ ] Apply honey to a clean face with your fingertips

- ☐ Leave on skin for 10-20 minutes
- ☐ Wash off with warm water and pat dry gently with a towel
- ☐ Apply your favorite toner, serum, and moisturizer

__Note:__ Any honey will do, but local or raw honey will provide the most skin benefits — just make sure it's 100% pure honey and not something diluted with additional components.

<u>Here are three simple adjustments to this basic recipe if you wish to tweak it:</u>

Nourishing: Spirulina + Honey Face Mask

Ingredients

- ☐ 3 tbsp honey
- ☐ 1 tbsp organic spirulina powder

- Optional essential oils – strongly suggested to cover the strong natural aroma of the spirulina
- ½ drops total of any combination of the following: orange, geranium, frankincense, lavender, rose (I'm a big fan of essential oils, so I use a few drops of each)

Instructions

- Start my by mixing all of the ingredients in a small bowl until a thick paste forms.
- To emulsify, place a small quantity in the palm of your hand and add a few drops of water.
- Apply with your fingers to a clean face

- ☐ Let dry and rest on skin for 10-20 minutes
- ☐ Wash off and pat dry gently
- ☐ Follow with your preferred toner, serum, and moisturizer
- ☐ Store any unused mask in a glass container in the fridge for up to 1 month.

Notes:

- ☐ This mask differs from the other two in that it forms a concentration that must be diluted with water before use.
- ☐ Do not add the water until you are ready to use it.
- ☐ The concentrate will harden up in the fridge, so use a spoon to get it out and add warm water to it. Products containing water require

preservatives, so simply take out what you need and add water to the palm of your hand. It'll soften up quickly.

Brightening: Pumpkin and Orange Face Mask

Ingredients

- [ ] 1 1/2 tbs pumpkin (the unsweetened sort that comes in a can)
- [ ] 1 ½ tbs honey
- [ ] 3-5 drops essential oils, try orange essential oil for brightening

Instructions

- [ ] Mix the ingredients in any container
- [ ] Apply to a clean face with your fingers or a brush

- ☐ Let dry and keep on skin for 10-20 minutes (the mask will stay wet and will not dry like a clay mask)
- ☐ Wash off and gently pat dry
- ☐ After that, apply your preferred toner, serum, and moisturizer.
- ☐ If there's any unused mask, keep in the refrigerator for a week.

If you wish to use this recipe a few times a week, double or triple the recipe, make a small batch and use it for a little self-care during the week, as required.

Clarifying: Bentonite Clay + Acv Face Mask

Ingredients

- ☐ 1 tablespoon bentonite clay

- [ ] 2 tablespoons apple cider vinegar (or water if you have sensitive skin)
- [ ] 1 tablespoon honey
- [ ] 3-5 drops essential oils Try rosemary, clary sage, blue tansy, copaiba, or tea tree oil for clarifying.

Instructions

- [ ] Combine clay and liquid (ACV or water) in a small bowl
- [ ] Stir in the honey until well mixed
- [ ] Apply to clean face using your fingers
- [ ] Then , leave on skin for 10-20 minutes (because it's a clay mask, you'll feel it tighten on your skin and see it change to a lighter color, this is normal)

⬜ Wash off and gently pat dry

NOTE: This mask also works great without the honey, so if you're pressed for time, simply blend those two components in the palm of your hand and apply directly.

Benefits Of Facial Masks

Facial masks are one of the simplest ways to achieve healthy, supple skin in a matter of minutes. Facial masks are developed for various skin and age types, and they come with a number of options and cosmetic features. The use of a face mask is quick and easy, and it provides numerous benefits. It is strongly advised that you incorporate it into your skin care routine.

Here are my top five benefits of wearing a face mask:

- **Refines skin pores**: Using a face mask will help you achieve cleaner skin and refined pores. It deep cleanses the pores, removing dead skin cells, metabolic wastes, and greasy substances that might clog them.

- **Increases hydration**: A face mask can also add moisture and hydration to dry or parched skin. The water in the mask penetrates deep into the epidermis of the skin, softening it and increasing its flexibility. It is easier to apply correct makeup when the skin is hydrated and thoroughly moisturized. It also provides the skin a more plump and youthful appearance.

- **Reduces fine lines**: Using face masks on a regular basis will help to minimize the indicators of aging such as fine lines, wrinkles, brown spots, and so on. You will also notice that your skin is softer and smoother.

- **Evens out skin tone**: Face masks are also intended to reduce hyperpigmentation and provide you with more even skin tone and texture. It also stimulates sweat gland secretion, which increases the skin's oxygen content.

- **Firmer skin**: Loose skin might make you appear older than your actual age. The problem of loose skin can be readily treated by using face masks on a regular basis. Certain types of face masks help to boost collagen formation and fight off free radical damage, resulting in firmer, tighter, and more youthful-looking skin over time.

Aside from the cosmetic benefits listed above, applying a face mask also helps you relax. While your face mask is functioning, you have time to rest. This will help you de-stress, which will make you look and feel better.

When considering the benefits of applying a face mask, it is safe to say that it is well worth the time and effort to incorporate it into your weekly beauty skin care routine.

Using Steam In Place Of Scrubs And Masks

Looking for a low-cost solution to improve your skin care routine? Facial steaming is a DIY skin care procedure that cleanses, nourishes, and feels luxurious.

Continue reading to learn how to achieve a gorgeous glow by utilizing steam instead of scrubbing and masks.

What Effect Does Steaming Have On Your Skin?

- **It's purifying** -- Steam opens your pores and aids in the removal of dirt accumulation for a more thorough wash. Blackheads are also softened when your pores are opened, making them easier to eliminate.

- **It improves circulation** -- Warm steam in combination with increased sweating dilates and enhances circulation in your blood vessels. This blood flow growth feeds your skin and oxygenates it. The end result is a healthy, natural glow.

- **It causes acne-causing bacteria and cells to be released** -- Opening your pores allows dead skin cells, germs, and other pollutants that clog your pores and contribute to acne to be released.

- **It expel trapped sebum** -- Your sebaceous glands create this naturally occurring oil to lubricate your skin and hair. When sebum becomes trapped underneath the surface of your skin, it produces a breeding ground for bacteria, resulting in acne and blackheads.

- **It has a moisturizing effect** -- Steam hydrates the skin by increasing oil production, which naturally moisturizes the face.

- **It improves the absorption of skin care products** -- Steam enhances skin permeability, allowing it to absorb topicals more effectively. This means that skin care products applied after a steam will give you more bang for your cash.

- **It stimulates the production of collagen and elastin** -- The increased blood flow that occurs during a steam facial encourages the synthesis of collagen and elastin. As a result, the skin appears firmer and younger.

- **It's calming** -- The sensation of warm steam on your face is soothing. Aromatherapy using herbs or essential oils can take your steam session to a whole new level of relaxation.

- **It relieves sinus congestion** -- Steam can help reduce sinus congestion and headaches, which are frequently associated with it. Adding essential oils to your steam might enhance the effect.

- **It is reasonably priced and easily accessible** -- You don't have to spend a lot of money on a steam facial at a spa to reap the benefits; you can do it at home with products you already have.

Various Strategies To Try

You may enjoy this adaptable skin treatment in a variety of ways at home. It can be as simple and free or as opulent and expensive as you and your wallet desire.

<u>Each strategy is described in detail below:</u>

- **To steam over a hot water bowl or sink**

  1. Take a large fluffy towel and choose a comfortable location. Because comfort is important, if you're doing this over a sink, choose a chair or stool with the appropriate height. If all else fails, a bowl on a table is your best hope.

  2. Pull your hair back from your face and cleanse with a gentle

exfoliating cleanser. Don't forget to scrub your neck as well.

3. In a kettle or saucepan, bring 4 to 6 cups of water to a boil, depending on the size of the sink or bowl.

4. Add a few herbs and stir as soon as the water starts boiling.

5. Reduce the heat to low, cover, and leave to simmer for 2 to 3 minutes. Pour into a sink or bowl with care. If you're using essential oils, add a few drops to the water now.

6. Throw a towel over your head, and lift your face 6 inches above water while sitting.

7. Raise or lower your head for more or less heat, and lift a

towel corner to cool off as necessary.

8. Steam your face for 5–10 minutes.

Using warm towels to steam

1. Take out a hand towel and turn on the hot water faucet. Fill your sink or basin with plenty of warm water to dip your towel, then put it in your herbs.

2. Pull your hair back from your face and cleanse your face and neck with a gentle exfoliating cleanser.

3. Soak your towel in hot water and wring it out until it is moist.

4. Just sit down or lie down on a convenient chair. Put the towel over your face, holding each corner to the middle of your brow.

5. Adjust the towel to cover your complete face, including your eyes, with only your nose poking through. Take 5 minutes to unwind.

To steam with a facial steamer at home

1. Follow the instructions on your face steamer, filling it up as indicated. Place it near an outlet on a table so you can plug it in. It will take a few minutes for the steam to start evaporating.

2. Pull your hair back from your face and wash your face with a gentle exfoliating cleanser.

3. Take a seat, get comfortable, and place your face inside the cone attachment, keeping your face 5 to 10 inches away as directed in the steamer's instruction booklet.

4. Take a 1-minute gap between 2 or 3 minutes of steam to see how your skin reacts to the steam.

How to Select a Base

The base you use at the end of the day to heat your face won't make steaming less useful, although some bases can bring further benefits.

<u>It all comes down to personal preference and financial constraints:</u>

- **Tap water** -- You can't really go wrong with tap water because it's easily accessible and free.

- **Spring or distilled water** -- You might also use distilled or spring water, however there is no evidence that one is better for steaming than the other.

- ☐ **Tea** -- Beauty teas include antioxidants, which are beneficial to your health from the inside out. They're also claimed to aid in the removal of toxins from your body. When applied topically, green tea and other polyphenol-containing beverages have been shown in studies to have anti-aging and protective properties.

How to Include Herbs and Oils

Adding dry herbs and essential oils to your steam may provide additional advantages. Certain herbs are regarded to be more useful for certain skin types than others. Depending on what you're looking for, several essential oils and herbs are known to provide a relaxing or stimulating effect.

Herbs

- **Chamomile** -- has been shown in research to aid with skin irritation and dermatitis, making it suitable for all skin types, especially sensitive skin.

- **Rosemary** -- This fragrant plant may be beneficial to those with oily skin.

Oils

- **Lavender** -- This plant is beneficial for dry skin and dermatitis, and it also has aromatherapy properties.

- **Geranium** -- **This** geranium flower oil is a natural astringent that tightens and tones the skin.

- **Eucalyptus** -- This is an excellent alternative if you have acne or are congested.

- **Orange** -- In addition to having uplifting aromatherapy effects, orange may aid with blocked pores and a dull complexion.

General Hints And Techniques

Here are some pointers to help you make the most of face steaming.

Preparation

- **Stay hydrated** -- Drinking water before exposing yourself to any type of heat is a good idea, so do so before you begin.
- **Do a cleanse** -- Wash your face with a light cleanser that includes an exfoliant so that your skin is ready to savor the benefits of steaming.

During The Steam

- Keep your eyes closed -- You'll be more comfortable, you won't risk irriting your eyes, and your eyelids will benefit from the steam.

- You do not want to come close to the bowl or sink too closely since you might get burnt. Keep your face 6-10 inches from the screen. Pay attention to your skin and do what feels right.

- When using a facial steamer, follow the manufacturer's instructions -- Read the instruction manual and use your facial steamer according to the directions.

Immediately after

- **Rinse and wipe dry with lukewarm water --** You don't want to aggravate your skin by wiping it with a cloth because it will be more sensitive.

- **Apply a moisturizing moisturizer or serum to your skin --** After a steam, the effects of your moisturizer or serum will be intensified, so use something nourishing. If you want younger-looking skin, now is the time to use an anti-aging cream.

- **Gently massage your face** -- What better way to cap off a soothing face steam than with a gentle face massage? Massage your forehead, cheeks, and neck in upward strokes with your fingers. Unless you have oily or sensitive skin, a small amount of face oil can be used to improve your massage.

Risks And Potential Adverse Effects

Because steam can inflict severe burns, it is critical to remain a safe distance from the source of the steam. If you're using a damp towel to steam your face, be sure it's warm, not hot.

If you have rosacea, you should avoid heating your face. Heat causes blood vessels to dilate, which contributes to redness.

Though steaming helps moisturize the skin, those with extremely dry skin or eczema should exercise extreme caution. To avoid irritation, keep steam sessions to a few minutes.

CHAPTER 3: MAKING MOISTURIZERS

When you look at the ingredients list of any natural moisturizer, you will see two key elements: oil (which may be described as a number of various oils and butter) and water.

Isn't it simple to combine oil and water?

However, the old saying holds true: oil and water do not mix. So a third ingredient, an emulsifier, is required to assist the oil and water join and stay together.

Making your own moisturising lotion is quick and easy, far cheaper than buying natural moisturizers, and much better for your skin than commercial moisturizers that contain a slew of questionable chemicals.

Recipe For Moisturizers For Dry Skin

Learn how to prepare the best body moisturizer recipes for dry skin treatment if you have dry skin. These natural skin care recipes for dry skin creams, oils, lotions, and balms are simple home remedies. They are free of the ingredients you don't want in your normal skin care regimen, so they don't aggravate dry skin further. Furthermore, they will not aggravate irritated skin if you have sensitive skin that is prone to adverse responses to over-the-counter body moisturizers.

Body Moisturizer Oil Recipes

Another technique to make a homemade body moisturizer is to combine carrier oils with skin-nourishing and moisturizing characteristics. These finest body moisturizer oil recipes are made with a mixture of moisturizing oils with unique qualities that do not leave skin feeling greasy after application. They are quick and simple to use because you simply spritz them on and massage them into dry skin for immediate relief.

DIY Dry Skin Body Oil Recipe

Ingredients

- 4 ounces hemp seed oil
- 1.5 ounces argan oil
- 2 oz. jojoba oil
- 5 oz. rosehip seed oil or tamanu oil
- 1 ml vitamin E oil
- 1/2 ml rosemary extract
- 2 ml optional essential oil

Weigh your carrier oils in a glass measuring cup using a digital kitchen scale. Next, measure out the vitamin E and rosemary extract with a different plastic transfer pipette for each oil and add to the container of oils. You can also add up to 2 ml of your preferred essential oil(s) or 4 ml of your preferred fragrance oil if desired.

After bathing, massage this body oil all over your body, focusing on the regions that require the greatest attention. Apply a natural body butter or salve to areas afflicted by itchy, dry skin or eczema.

Body Moisturizing Salve And Essential Oils Recipe

This essential oil-infused healing salve recipe is ideal for winter skin treatment.

This natural body moisturizer moisturizes and protects skin with all natural ingredients, including a simple mixture of warming essential oils to assist improve circulation and reduce inflammation, and can be used as a soothing salve for dry hands. Because of the basic essential oil mixture, it is especially beneficial if you have tight joints, sore muscles, or arthritis. This healing hand salve recipe is a one-of-a-kind two-in-one treatment that provides both dry skin treatment and pain alleviation without the use of several treatments. It also naturally warms cold hands.

DIY Healing Salve Recipe

Ingredients

- ☐ 1 oz. baobab oil
- ☐ 5 oz. shea nut oil

- ☐ 5 oz. beeswax pastilles
- ☐ 1-2 drops vitamin E oil
- ☐ 9 mL blood orange essential oil
- ☐ 6 mL ginger essential oil

Instructions

1. In a double boiler, combine the baobab oil, shea nut oil, and beeswax.

2. When the chocolate has melted, remove it from the fire. Then, to the healing hand salve, add the vitamin E oil and essential oils. To blend, stir everything together.

3. Pour the healing salve into a 2 oz. amber glass container that has been sterilized. Allow to cool completely before using.

Body Moisturizer Lotion Recipe

If you have acne-prone or mixed skin, applying heavy body moisturizers may exacerbate breakouts. You can moisturize without worry if you use a lotion to treat dry skin. Lotion formulations are typically produced with a significant amount of water or milk to moisturize skin. As a result, they are frequently more lightweight than body creams, which contain little water, or body butters, which contain no water. So, they're less likely to block pores.

Because body lotions contain water, an emulsifier is required to prevent the oil and water from separating. This, paired with controlled mixing temperatures, ensures the optimum lotion.

However, because body lotions contain water, they will require a preservative to prevent bacteria, mold, and other germs from forming and causing skin illnesses. If you don't want to use preservatives but still want to produce homemade body lotions, I propose starting with a lotion base that may then be scented with essential oils or a fragrance oil to your preferences.

DIY Cooling Cucumber Lotion Recipe

Ingredients

- 1 cucumber
- 1/4 cup coconut milk
- 1/4 cup aloe vera juice

Instructions

To juice the cucumber, coarsely shred it and drain it through a cheesecloth or strainer over a bowl. Push the cucumber to get the liquid out. One cucumber yielded about a cup of juice.

Pour into a jar with a cover and add the coconut milk and aloe vera. Shake well to mix. Store in the refrigerator.

Use a spray bottle to apply to the skin, or moisten a washcloth and apply to irritated regions.

Recipe for moisturizers for oily skin

Oily skin is considered to be one of the most difficult skin types to manage to appear healthy and young. Because it secretes extra oils, many people avoid moisturizing and end up with more acne and dark patches as a result. Some moisturizers cause breakouts because they include a lot of pollutants and chemicals, which is why you should always be careful about what you put on your skin. Homemade moisturizers for oily skin are simple to customize based on your skin type and budget.

Another common misconception is that moisturizers for oily skin make your skin more oily and greasy, making it more prone to acne and having a dull appearance. Not all oils, however, regulate sebum secretion, decreasing acne production and providing you with healthy, glowing skin in exchange.

Milk and Olive Oil

Ingredients

- 1/4 quarter cup of fresh milk
- 2-3 tablespoons extra virgin olive oil
- 2-3 tablespoons lemon juice

Instructions

Mix all of the ingredients together, then apply to your face with a cotton ball and wait for it to dry; this is one of the best moisturizers for oily skin that does not cause breakouts. This is due to the fact that milk contains lactic acid, which has soothing and calming effects and is also a wonderful anti-bacterial agent.

Olive Oil is an anti-microbial natural source that destructs acne-causing bacteria, while lemon juice controls oil secretion to eliminate greasiness that gives an unsatisfactory look. It is best to apply these sorts of facial moisturizers for oily skin at night because olive oil might develop dark spots if exposed to sunlight.

Jojoba oil Moisturizer

Ingredients

- ☐ 1 tsp Jojoba oil
- ☐ 3 drops essential oil of Frankincense
- ☐ 3 drops essential lavender oil

Instructions

Jojoba oil is one of the best oily skin moisturizers since it is comparable to skin sebum itself, it offers an overall equilibrium between the oil yields and a healthy appearance for your skin. Jojoba oil is very easily absorbed by the skin, thus there is no greasiness. You can use it alone or construct an oil mixture moisturizer.

Frankincense essential oil contains anti-inflammatory and anti-bacterial characteristics, making it an effective acne treatment. It is also well-known for its ability to reduce scars and wrinkles, making it one of the greatest moisturizers for oily skin. It is a little pricey, so if you can't afford it, leave it out of the blend. Lavender essential oil has antibacterial characteristics that assist to minimize any redness or irritation caused by acne.

Mix all of the ingredients in a small dropper and begin applying a few drops to your face. You can apply the moisturizer whenever you want, but it is best to apply at night to reap the greatest benefits.

Shea Butter and Jojoba Oil

Ingredients

- 1/8 Cup of Jojoba oil
- 1/4 Cup of Shea Butter

Instructions

To begin, melt the shea butter in a steam bath and add the jojoba oil when it becomes liquid. Mix the liquid thoroughly and place it in the fridge for approximately an hour till it solidifies. Remove from the fridge and add a few drops of any essential oil you prefer, then whip it until it turns into a creamy texture before packing it in a nice mason jar.

Shea butter is strong in vitamin A, E and fatty acids and is not curative, so pores are not blocked and breakouts are not caused, making the shea butter one of the best moisturizers for skin with an oily appearance.

This is an excellent winter moisturizer that also works well on combination skin and requires only a tiny quantity.

Aloe Vera Moisturizer

Ingredients

- ☐ 1/4 Cup of Jojoba oil
- ☐ 1/4 Cup of Aloe vera gel
- ☐ 3 drops essential oil of rose

Instructions

In a container of your choice, combine all the ingredients and place them in a fridge; remember to shake before using because aloe solidifies in low heat. It is a terrific summer moisturizer that you may use at any time because it is light on your skin and controls sebum secretion, giving you healthy-looking skin.

This is due to the fact that rose essential oil cleans your skin and removes all dirt, whereas aloe vera shrinks acne and heals scars due to its anti-inflammatory and antioxidant content, which keeps your skin firm without any greasiness, making it one of the most effective moisturizers for oily skin.

Recipe for moisturizer combination skin

If you have combination skin that is oily in particular areas (such as your T-zone), it could be due to a lack of moisture or overuse of stripping products. Natural oils quickly infiltrate the pores and assist the skin in resuming its own moisture production, which is the ultimate goal. When it comes to oils, I recommend soft, moisturizing hazelnut oil (which has astringent characteristics), hydrating, collagen-boosting avocado oil, and sesame and jojoba oil, both of which are light and work wonders to keep microorganisms at away on the surface of your skin.

Ingredients

- [ ] 1 tablespoon avocado oil
- [ ] 1 tablespoon hazelnut oil
- [ ] 1 tablespoon sesame oil (or jojoba oil)

Instructions

1. Mix the oils together. Fill a tiny dropper bottle halfway with all three oils, screw on the cap, and shake to combine.
2. It's as simple as that. Keep in mind that this recipe only yields ½ servings, so feel free to double it if you need more.

Aside from the cost, because it's an oil moisturizer rather than a solid lotion or cream, you're less likely to bring bacteria into the bottle because you can disseminate the mix with a dropper. Even so, I recommend using it within six months of making it.

3. When using the formula, rub it into your face to activate the oils. Furthermore, it is best used at night; if you intend to wear makeup, wash it off first. However, if you adore a dewy complexion, another alternative is to use simply a drop or two and pat it into your skin, eliminating any excess with a towel.

Benefits Of Moisturizing

Daily moisturizing is one of the simplest ways to make the skin look the finest. Continue reading to learn more about the benefits of moisturizing your skin:

- **Appear Younger** – Incorporating a high quality moisturizer into your daily regimen is one of the best methods to prevent wrinkles and keep your skin radiant and fresh. Keeping your skin moist, especially during the colder months, can greatly improve the texture and appearance.

- **Prevent Dryness** - Using a moisturizer on a daily basis can avoid your skin from becoming dry and flaky. Nothing is more unpleasant than uneven skin that is discolored and patchy. Provide your skin with the moisturizing and emulsifying elements it needs to look and feel its best for a smooth, touchable face and an even complexion.

- **Fight Acne** - When your skin dries out, your glands receive a signal that it is time to generate additional sebum, which can clog your pores and trigger breakouts. It may seem paradoxical, but keeping your face hydrated is essential for keeping acne at bay and preventing it from becoming excessively oily.

- **Sun Protection** - These days, even during the cooler months, medical professionals advocate a daily dose of SPF. You can maintain your skin healthy and battle cancer at the same time by finding a moisturizer that has sun protection.

- **Save Sensitive Skin** - Redness, eczema, and itchy spots are all too prevalent for those of us with sensitive skin. Choose a moisturizer that has skin-calming components such as chamomile and aloe vera to keep your face protected from the weather and looking its best.

CHAPTER 4: REDUCING WRINKLES

Wrinkles are the body's way of displaying the fact that you are becoming older. Everyone gets wrinkles as they get older. Nonetheless, some people get wrinkles years or decades before their contemporaries. There are numerous elements that can influence the formation of wrinkles in your skin. By avoiding those causes, you can prevent the early formation of wrinkles. Nobody wants those lines in their skin because they are indication that their body is aging.

At Home Ways To Reduce Wrinkles

There are numerous home cures for facial wrinkles available that are simply ready to be applied. Continue reading if you have no idea what I'm talking about.

Today, the cosmetics sector is one of the most important markets on the planet. A large number of people are looking for solutions to minimize wrinkles, and it can be difficult to sort through all of the advertising and hoopla.

Here are a few basic home remedies for drastically reducing wrinkles:

Water

Lots of water is the best and simplest home cure for anti-wrinkle skin care. Water is recognized for eliminating toxins from the body, therefore drinking 8 to 10 glasses of water every day will help. Make sure you don't drink all of your water at once, but rather break it up throughout the day and consume at least 2 to 3 liters at the end of the day.

Face Pack

Another anti-wrinkle skin care tip is to construct your own face pack from components found in your kitchen. <u>To make the face pack, you'll need the following items:</u>

- ☐ Cucumber Juice
- ☐ 1 egg white
- ☐ 1 tablespoon honey
- ☐ 1 tablespoon brandy

Combine these four ingredients, apply to your face, and let on for ten to fifteen minutes before rinsing with Luke warm water.

Homemade face packs are really effective, and you will notice an immediate improvement in the radiance of your skin.

Moisturizers and oils

Applying coconut oil or pure castor oil to your skin once a night also aids in the softening and hydration of the skin. This can aid in the prevention of wrinkles. A light moisturizing cream is also beneficial.

Apple and Pineapple Juice

When apple and pineapple juice is applied to the skin on a daily basis, it helps to reduce wrinkles. Allow it to sink for 10 to 15 minutes before rinsing with warm water.

Powdered turmeric

Turmeric powder also has a remarkable anti-aging impact on the skin, especially when combined with sugarcane juice.

Skin Massage

Massage your skin in a circular motion from the neck up until you reach the forehead is another cure that is highly beneficial to the skin. We all require some form of exercise, thus exercising our faces is essential. Massaging the face also aids in drawing blood to the face.

Avocado

Avocado's oil content also contributes to the appearance of vibrant, youthful skin. You can chop the fruit into slices and apply the pulp or slices on your face for a natural anti-aging effect. This is a really vital and beneficial skin care solution. Consuming foods high in fiber and vitamin C is essential for anti-wrinkle skin care.

Lemon Juice

A dab of lemon juice applied to your face every morning when you wake up is very significant in eliminating wrinkles. Dab lemon on your skin, let it for 15 minutes, and then rinse off.

Natural Products To Reduce Wrinkles

Superfoods

Superfoods are foods that are high in health-promoting ingredients. Many superfoods appear to reduce wrinkles and improve general health.

<u>Many superfoods, including those listed below, may help minimize the appearance of wrinkles:</u>

- ☐ Avocados
- ☐ Artichokes
- ☐ Cinnamon
- ☐ Egg whites
- ☐ Chia seeds
- ☐ Miso
- ☐ Ginger
- ☐ Oatmeal
- ☐ Sardines
- ☐ Tomatoes
- ☐ Salmon
- ☐ Sweet potatoes

Essential oils

Applying essential oils blended with a carrier oil on wrinkles may help minimize their appearance. Essential oils are frequently used in precise combinations to cure skin without causing irritation, provided they are diluted with a carrier oil.

<u>When used in various combinations with a carrier, the following essential oils may help improve the look of wrinkles:</u>

- ☐ Carrot seed
- ☐ Clary sage
- ☐ Argan
- ☐ Geranium
- ☐ Frankincense
- ☐ Grapeseed
- ☐ Helichrysum
- ☐ Jojoba

- ☐ Lavender
- ☐ Ylang-ylang
- ☐ Rosemary
- ☐ Pomegranate
- ☐ Rose
- ☐ Sandalwood
- ☐ Neroli

Minerals

Minerals, like vitamins, are micronutrients contained in meals that your body requires in little amounts. Minerals in the skin help to filter sunlight, promote healing, and prevent harm.

Zinc and selenium are two nutrients that are particularly beneficial to skin health. A topical lotion containing zinc and selenium can help to prevent the skin from sun damage that creates wrinkles by blocking some UV rays.

Selenium-containing dietary supplements may have the same protective effects. However, if you eat a healthy diet, you should be getting enough zinc and selenium.

<u>Zinc may be found in the following foods:</u>

- ☐ Oysters
- ☐ Beans
- ☐ Almonds
- ☐ Oatmeal
- ☐ Peas
- ☐ Cheese

<u>Foods high in selenium include:</u>

- ☐ Sunflower seeds
- ☐ Yogurt

- ☐ Spinach
- ☐ Oatmeal
- ☐ Bananas

Too much zinc and selenium can be harmful to your health, so consult your doctor before adding supplements to your diet.

CHAPTER 5: TREATING ACNE AND SCARS

If you've battled acne and come out on top, it may feel like the struggle is over. However, many blemishes leave a scar on your skin long after the breakout has healed. Pitted scars and red pigmentation patches can remain for months – even years – but there are techniques you can use to smooth your way back to bright, even skin, which I'll teach you in this chapter.

At Home Ways To Treat Acne

Acne has become so common among teenagers and adults that many specialists throughout the world charge exorbitant fees for acne treatment. It's not even funny to check around for advanced acne treatment price ranges. The treatment of this illness should not be prohibitively expensive.

You can, however, do it on your own by employing powerful acne home treatments. <u>The following steps are widely recommended by skin experts and can be performed safely at home:</u>

1. Washing your face on a daily basis should be a habit. Many people believe that only women should do this because of the makeup they wear during the day, but it is essential for everyone, including guys. Acne is more likely in people who do not wash their faces at night. Consider sleeping with dirt and bacteria swimming about your face.

1. You should also practice this during the day if you have the opportunity. If you manage to sneak into the restroom during lunch, wash your face with water and gently dry it with a tissue or a towel.

2. Fill your glass with water. You are well aware of the importance of water in your system. Fluids not only improve skin tone, but they also wash away particles and impurities, resulting in cleaner, healthier skin. Adults should drink at least 10 glasses of water every day.

3. Make use of vitamin E. This sort of vitamin is popular among skin care enthusiasts due to its exfoliating and rejuvenating properties. Vitamin E can be found in lotion or oil form at

your local grocery or health shop. Simply apply it immediately to the affected area and leave it on overnight. Another approach to get vitamin E into your system is to take a vitamin E tablet once a day. Look for well-known brands to ensure that you're only getting pure vitamin E and nothing else.

4. Just keep your hands away from your face. This is a simple guideline, but you are certain to commit an error unconsciously. It is important to keep alcohol on hand at all times so that you can wash your hands with it. Other acne home cures include avoid using oily hair products or greasy make-up to reduce oil contact on your face.

Natural Solutions For Acne

Acne can be obstinate and appear at inconvenient times. The good news is that retail and prescription medicinal products can help remove pimples and prevent future outbursts. The bad news is that several acne treatments might cause redness, discolouration, or dryness. As a result, some people opt to treat acne at home with natural remedies:

- **Create a honey-cinnamon mask**

Honey and cinnamon have the capacity to fight bacteria and reduce inflammation, both of which contribute to acne.

Instructions

1. Make a paste with 2 tablespoons of honey and 1 teaspoon cinnamon.

2. After cleaning your skin, apply the mask and leave it on for 10–15 minutes.

3. Rinse the mask thoroughly and massage your skin dry.

- **Spot treat with tea tree oil**

Tea tree oil has a well-known capacity to kill microorganisms and minimize skin inflammation.

Instructions

1. Combine 1 part tea tree oil and 9 parts water.

2. Dip a cotton swab into the solution and dab it on the afflicted regions.

3. If desired, apply moisturizer.

4. Repeat this method 1–2 times each day, if necessary.

- **Use green tea to moisturize your skin**

Green tea includes a lot of antioxidants to keep you healthy. It may also aid in the reduction of acne. This is most likely due to the polyphenols in green tea, which help combat germs and reduce inflammation, both of which are major causes of acne.

Instructions

1. Steep green tea for 3–4 minutes in boiling water.
2. Set aside the tea to cool.
3. Apply the tea to your skin with a cotton ball or spritz it on with a spray bottle.

4. Allow it to dry before rinsing with water and patting your skin dry.

- **Use witch hazel**

Witch hazel contains tannins, which are antibacterial and anti-inflammatory in nature. As a result, it is used to treat a wide variety of skin disorders, including dandruff, eczema, varicose veins, burns, bruises, bug bites, and acne.

Instructions

1. In a small saucepan, combine 1 tablespoon witch hazel bark and 1 cup water.
2. Soak the witch hazel in water for 30 minutes before bringing it to a boil on the burner.
3. Reduce to a low heat and cook for 10 minutes, covered.

4. Remove the mixture from the heat and set aside for 10 minutes.

5. Strain the liquid and keep it in a well sealed jar.

6. Apply with a cotton ball to clean skin 1–2 times a day, or as desired.

- **Use aloe vera to moisturize**

Aloe vera is a tropical plant that produces a transparent gel from its leaves. The gel is frequently incorporated into lotions, creams, ointments, and soaps.

It is often used to treat skin diseases such as abrasions, rashes, burns, and others. Aloe vera gel can help heal the injuries, treat burns and reduce inflammations when applied to the skin. Aloe vera includes salicylic acid and sulfur, both of which are commonly used in the treatment of acne.

Instructions

1. Scrape the gel off of the aloe plant with a spoon.
2. As a moisturizer, apply the gel immediately to clean skin.
3. Repeat 1–2 times daily, or as needed.

At Home Way To Fix Scars

Scars can form as a result of an injury, burns, acne, pimples, bug bites, chickenpox, or surgery. They have the potential to tarnish your skin and leave lasting markings on your face and/or body. Although some portions of the body are not visible, having these scars on places such as the face can be humiliating and difficult to deal with.

While these scars do not completely disappear, they do fade with time. In this book, I've included a variety of home remedies that can help speed up scar lightening and make them less visible. <u>Look at this:</u>

- **Lime**

Lemons contain a high concentration of bioactive chemicals that have antioxidant capabilities. These can help restore your skin and lessen the appearance of scars caused by acne, pimples, or zits.

Ingredients

- ☐ 3–4 tsp lemon juice
- ☐ Cotton ball

Instructions

1. Cleanse the skin around the scar.
2. Dab the afflicted region with a cotton ball dipped in lemon juice.
3. Leave it on approximately 10 minutes before rinsing.
4. Apply sunscreen after washing off the lemon juice if you intend to go outside in the sun.

How Often Should You Do This?

This should be done 2-3 times per day.

NOTE: *Because lemon juice can generate a stinging feeling on your skin, you should only use it if you are not sensitive to it.*

- **Bees**

Raw honey has long been used to treat scars. It includes bioactive chemicals that promote tissue regeneration and can help with wound healing. Baking soda serves as an exfoliator and aids in scar whitening.

Ingredients

- 1 tsp raw honey
- 1 tsp baking soda
- A small towel
- Hot water

Instructions

1. Combine the raw honey and baking soda in a mixing bowl.
2. Apply the mixture on the scar for 3-5 minutes.
3. Place a heated towel over the affected region. Wipe the area clean once the cloth has cooled.

How Often Should You Do This?

Do this at least twice a day.

- **Onion**

Onions have anti-inflammatory effects as well as the ability to prevent collagen formation, which aids in the fading of scars.

Ingredients

- The juice of an onion

Instructions

1. Peel and grate an onion, then squeeze out some fresh onion juice.
2. Apply immediately to the scar and let it to dry naturally.
3. After 15 minutes, rinse thoroughly.

How Often Should You Do This?

This can be done 3-4 times a day.

NOTE: *Remember to keep your skin hydrated in between onion juice applications.*

- **Aloe Vera Gel**

Aloe vera gel has anti-inflammatory properties. This may aid in the reduction of skin irritation and scarring, as well as the regeneration of new skin cells.

Ingredients

- Aloe vera gel

Instructions

1. Apply freshly extracted aloe vera gel or an organic store-bought aloe vera gel on the scars. Massage it in completely.
2. Do not rinse it.

How Often Should You Do This?

Reapply 2-3 times per day.

- **Gooseberry**

Gooseberry is high in vitamin C, which may aid in scar reduction. Because of its tyrosinase inhibiting activity, it can help to minimize the appearance of scars. As a result, it may lessen pre-existing scars while also preventing the production of new ones.

Ingredients

- Gooseberry powder
- Olive oil

Instructions

1. Combine enough gooseberry powder and olive oil to make a smooth paste to cover the affected region.
2. Apply as a face mask and leave on for 10-15 minutes.

3. Rinse with cold water.

How Often Should You Do This?

You can use this facial pack every other day.

- **Tea Tree Oil**

Tea tree oil contains phytochemicals that may aid in the progressive reduction of surgical and acne scars. It increases blood flow to the damaged area and protects it from infection.

Ingredients

- ☐ 1 teaspoon water or olive oil
- ☐ 2-3 drops tea tree oil

Instructions

1. Mix the tea tree essential oil with olive oil or water to dilute it.

2. Apply this oil to the scarred region.
3. Leave it on through the night.

How Often Should You Do This?

This should be done every night before going to bed.

Note: *Before using this remedy, perform a patch test because tea tree oil may produce an allergic reaction in some people.*

- **Coconut Oil**

Coconut oil includes phenolic compounds, antioxidants, and vitamins that can help skin cells and tissues thrive. This may aid in the removal of old scars, and its antibacterial characteristics may assist to prevent future breakouts.

Ingredients

☐ 1 tsp virgin coconut oil

Instructions

1. Rub the coconut oil between your palms to warm it.
2. Apply it to the scars with a cotton swab and leave it on overnight.

How Often Should You Do This?

Do this each night before you go to bed.

- **Potato Juice**

Potato juice is high in phytochemicals, which can be used to cleanse your skin and remove pigmentation or spots produced by acne and pimples. This gives your skin a refreshed and clearer appearance.

Ingredients

☐ 2 teaspoons potato juice

Instructions

1. Crush a raw potato to extract the juice.
2. Soak a cotton ball in the juice and dab it on the affected regions.
3. Leave it on for 10 minutes before rinsing it off.

How Often Should You Do This?

This juice should be applied 2-3 times per week.

- **Lavender Oil**

Lavender oil is antifungal, anti-inflammatory, and antibacterial in nature. This may aid in the battle against any inflammatory response to infections on your skin, as well as the healing of the damaged area and the elimination of scars over time.

Ingredients

- ☐ 2-3 drops lavender oil
- ☐ 1 teaspoon sweet almond oil

Instructions

1. Combine two to three drops of lavender oil and one teaspoon of sweet almond oil.
2. Apply the mixture to the afflicted regions with a cotton ball.
3. After 10 minutes, properly rinse your face.

How Often Should You Do This?

Do this 2-3 times every day.

- **Rosehip Oil**

Rosehip oil contains bioactive chemicals that have wound-healing effects. It has been discovered that it can hasten the shift of macrophage morphologies, which can assist heal scarring over time.

Ingredients

- 2-3 drops rosehip oil
- 1 teaspoon sweet almond oil

Instructions

1. Combine two to three drops rosehip oil and one teaspoon sweet almond oil.
2. Use the mixture to treat the damaged areas. Leave it on for the night.
3. Wash it off first thing in the morning.

How Often Should You Do This?

This can be done 2-3 times a day.

CHAPTER 6: LIGHT THERAPY

Light therapy is a non-invasive hand and face treatment that uses narrow band, non-thermal LED light energy to stimulate your body's natural cell processes, hence accelerating skin renewal and repair. It is indicated for skin rejuvenation, sun damage, acne, rosacea, eczema, psoriasis, dermatitis, sensitive and inflammatory disorders, wound healing and scarring, and anybody wishing to restore the radiance of their skin.

What Is the Purpose of Light Therapy?

LED Light Therapy is excellent in all facials for soothing any areas of inflammation and whitening the skin.

LED lights are supposed to penetrate your skin at different depths and induce various reactions in your skin, such as battling acne-causing germs, plumping skin, and reducing wrinkles, when used consistently and over time.

How Does Light Therapy Work?

LED Light Therapy employs visible light wavelengths with unique skin benefits. Healthy skin cells are impaired and unable to replenish themselves regularly as a result of aging, skin illnesses, or damage.

The skin uses light as an energy source to repair and rejuvenate damaged cells or, in the case of acne treatment, to kill germs. The energy increases collagen and elastin formation, improves circulation, and speeds up tissue repair. During the treatment, you will simply lie behind a light screen while the equipment performs all of the necessary functions.

Benefits Of Light Therapy

Light treatment for the skin helps alleviate skin diseases like rosacea and dermatitis while also speeding up wound healing. It is also used to treat acne and as an anti-aging device. Let's look at the advantages of various types of light therapy.

Benefits of red light therapy

Red light therapy has the following benefits:

- Promotes wound healing and tissue repair

- Improves hair growth in people with androgenic alopecia
- Aids in the short-term treatment of carpal tunnel syndrome
- Stimulates healing of slow-healing wounds such as diabetic foot ulcers
- Reduces psoriasis lesions

Benefits of green light therapy

Green light therapy has the following benefits:

- Lighter and smoother skin
- Reduction of spider veins and rosacea
- Reduction of hyperpigmentation and age spots
- Pain relief
- Wound healing
- Tissue repair

Benefits of yellow light therapy

Yellow light therapy has the following benefits:

- Alleviates UV radiation damage
- Drug-free alternative for skin redness and flushing
- Boosts lymphatic flow, which helps remove toxins from the targeted area
- Heals skin irritation and rosacea
- Reduces fine lines and wrinkles
- Reduces the appearance of tiny blood vessels on the nose/face
- Increases cellular growth

Benefits of blue light therapy

Blue light therapy has the following benefits:

- Effective for acne treatment

- ☐ Prevents oily skin
- ☐ Reduces blackheads
- ☐ Effective therapy for Eczema and Psoriasis

Purchasing Light Therapy Machines

Light treatment, also known as photobiomodulation or low-level laser therapy, is non-invasive, painless, and suited for all skin types. It does not require any rest or recuperation time.

When using a high-quality medical LED light therapy machine, a single LED light facial treatment can be completed in as little as 15 minutes. And it is supported by a slew of research that demonstrates clinical efficacy. A 2018 study, for example, discovered that LED treatment can improve the healing of severe skin burns.

How Do I Select the Most Appropriate LED Light Therapy Machine?

LED treatment machines are not all made equal.

For example, because of variances in the quality of the machine's constituent components, there can be significant changes in light output.

<u>When selecting the best LED therapy machine for your in home use, the following factors should be taken into account:</u>

- Wavelength
- Energy output (irradiance)
- Treatment coverage area
- Cooling
- Uniformity of distribution

☐ Manufacturer's depth of experience

As previously stated, the wavelengths of the emitted LEDs (measured in nanometers) will determine which indications you will be able to cure.

The device's power output (or, more precisely, its irradiance or light intensity) impacts how soon you can cure such indicators.

It is crucial to realize that LED wattage is not a reliable indicator of light output. An LED panel may consume twice as much electricity as another panel while emitting only a tenth of the light.

It is also critical to assess how successfully the LED is used in practice. To achieve optimal energy delivery for improved therapeutic outcomes, you'll want an

LED machine with uniform energy
distribution.

CONCLUSION

Developing A Routine For Your Face

If you have some more time to devote to skincare right now, it would be good to establish some healthier skin-care practices. Depending on your goals and what is essential to you, you can spend as much as an hour or as little as ten seconds on your skin, but for most individuals, a basic morning and evening regimen is best.

Morning Routine

- **Cleanse your face with a mild cleanser** -- In the morning, you generally don't have a lot of perspiration, grime, or other crud to remove. You're simply removing oil and dead skin cells to make way for newer, healthier cells. Look for products with few ingredients that are gentle on your skin.

- **Use any extras** - If you have a treatment for a specific skin issue (acne, eczema, psoriasis, etc.), use it after you wash. At this stage, you can also apply products such as antioxidants or antiaging serums.

- **Moisturize** - Use a decent moisturizer on a daily basis. This might range from a light water-based moisturizer to a heavier cream, depending on your skin type.

- **Sunscreen** – As long as the SPF is greater than 30, you can use a separate sunscreen or a moisturizer with built-in sunscreen.

- **Cosmetics -** If you wear cosmetics, you can apply them normally once your moisturizer and sunscreen have thoroughly absorbed into your skin. Beginning your cosmetic application with a primer can assist smooth the skin's surface and protect your skin from the potentially harsh ingredients in many makeup products.

Night Routine

- **Wash your face** - If you use makeup, make sure to completely remove it with a makeup remover, micellar water, or other solution that allows you to clear your skin of cosmetics without having to scrub and tug at your face. Then, wash your skin with a simple, gentle cleanser.

- **Exfoliate (on a regular basis)** – Exfoliate your skin once or twice a week to eliminate dead skin cells that can clog pores. Eczema sufferers may wish to avoid exfoliating or consult with their doctor about good choices for eczema-prone skin. Your dermatologist would advise you to avoid coarse exfoliating products regardless of your skin type because they can create unneeded aggravation. Instead, look for exfoliators or fine scrubs that contain enzymes or fruit acids.
- **Use extras** - If you wish to use an antiaging, retinoid, or a product

containing growth factors and peptides to promote cellular renewal, now is the time to do so. Many bedtime moisturizers and eye creams already contain these compounds, so you may wish to consult your dermatologist for a product recommendation that can provide these antiaging and antioxidant benefits without requiring an additional step.

- **Moisturize** - Use a thicker moisturizer at night to really saturate your skin while you sleep. After a day of stress and damage, thick, cream moisturizers and nighttime masks can help replenish your skin's hydration.

- **Get plenty of beauty sleep -** • Get a good night's sleep - Seriously. Get lots of sleep since your skin (and all of your cells) are restored and regenerated as you sleep.

Developing A Routine For Your Body

People frequently devote most of their time to caring for the skin on their faces. However, your skin is the greatest organ in your body and covers more than simply your face. As a result, caring for the rest of your body is equally as vital as caring for your skin.

Daily Routine For Whole Body

- **Clean up your act** – We all want to lather ourselves with those great smelling, perfumed body cleansers, but these products might cause skin irritation. Instead, for daily cleaning, use a light cleaner (preferably one that is natural). If you want to enjoy the interesting perfumes (as long as they don't hurt your skin), mix a small bit with your gentle cleanser to deliver the aroma without the unneeded chemicals.

- **Exfoliate the skin** — You should be conscious of your specific needs when exfoliating your face, and prevent over-exfoliation. Exfoliating once or twice a week is sufficient for practically everyone. Because the skin on your body is tougher than the skin on your face, you can use a scrub such as a sugar or salt-based alternative if your skin can withstand it. Furthermore, dry brushing the skin before showering may be beneficial in removing dead skin cells and stimulating circulation. Otherwise, consult your dermatologist about gentler exfoliation solutions for the entire body. Remember that places like the elbows, knees, and feet tend to have substantially more skin buildup, so exfoliate these regions with more care.

- **Stay hydrated** — Apply an excellent all-over body moisturizer immediately after bathing. This helps to catch and retain the advantages of the moisture surge you experience after showering. If you have extremely dry skin, you should apply a moisturizer at night as well, preferably a cream-based moisturizer rather than a lotion.

How Often Should You Give Yourself Facials?

Most people, both men and women, take care of their skin and hair only when they have a particular occasion to attend, such as a wedding, anniversaries, birthdays, reunions, or other gatherings. Women, in particular, go to great lengths in their beauty program to look their best, treating every minor cosmetic concern in order to display beautiful skin. But what about our skin the rest of the year? Most of the time, due to a lack of time, we disregard basic skin care procedures and convince ourselves that it is okay to do so.

Some people are hesitant to have a facial because they are unfamiliar with the fundamentals of skin care. However, in today's world, with pollution and stress levels at an all-time high, it frequently results in dull skin and skin degeneration. This makes it even more vital to pay attention to and care for your skin.

Facials should not be considered a once-in-a-while or special occasion treatment. They should be a part of your beauty routine on a daily basis. Yes, what you need in your twenties is nothing like what you might require in your forties or fifties; nonetheless, a facial is vital at both ages.

Other Beauty Tricks to Try

Some of the illusions you've heard over the years about DIY beauty are totally wrong. Whoever thought washing hair with beer was a good idea must have had one too many drinks, but there are some quick cures you can try at home that work. <u>Here are a few of my personal favorites:</u>

- **Step 1: After brushing your teeth, drink a large bottle of water**

Every night before bed, I fill a large glass bottle with water and place it on my bathroom counter. I drink it first thing in the morning, straight after brushing my teeth. Because I know that all of that breathing in and out through the night exhales a lot of moisture from my lungs. Consider how much water you can lose in an eight-hour period of breathing. We can't refill it while we sleep, so it's critical to rehydrate when we wake up. I immediately feel it after drinking the water from the bottle by my sink. I transform from a withered plant to one that has been revitalized by rain.

- **Step 2: Apply honey to your face as a mask**

Honey (raw honey, please) possesses antibacterial qualities and is particularly useful in treating acne-prone skin. Slather it on your face, leave it for 10 minutes, then wash it off with warm water, and you're done.

- **Step 3: Use baking soda to whiten your teeth**

Are you hesitant to spend money on pricey teeth whitening kits? For a healthy set of pearly whites, combine one tablespoon of baking soda with three drops of hydrogen peroxide and use it as toothpaste.

- **Step 4: Use hair conditioner to shave your legs**

Instead than purchasing a separate shaving foam, simply use hair conditioner. It's extremely moisturizing, making the hair softer and thus simpler to shave.

- **Step 5: Apply evening primrose oil to spots to help them heal faster**

Aside from the natural scar removal methods I mentioned previously. Primrose oil can aid in the healing of spots. Apply an evening primrose oil capsule to troubled areas to help them heal in half the time. It has anti-inflammatory effects that can significantly reduce the redness of painful regions. For optimal results, use it overnight and sleep in it.

- **Step 6: Always keep a pot of Vaseline nearby**

Petroleum jelly has a plethora of applications. One of my favorite things to do is slather it all over my feet, put on a pair of fuzzy socks, and go to bed. It's wonderful for avoiding color from coloring your skin if you colour your own hair; simply use it as a barrier around the hairline, ears, and neck. Finally, it can be used to tame wild brows.

- **Step 7: Lemon peel can be used to remove nail polish stains**

If your nails have been stained by black nail lacquer, simply massage some lemon peel over the troublesome area.

- **Step 8: Exfoliate with an orange**

Oranges' acid and Vitamin C content make them a good exfoliant. If you have no time for fantastic home-made potions and lotions, cut an orange half and use your knees and elbows.

- **Step 9: Shave your legs last**

If shaving causes bumpy or irritated legs, do it toward the end of your shower, when the warm water will have opened up your pores and the hair will be softer.

- **Step 10: Store your beauty products in the refrigerator**

Obviously, not all of them, but nail polishes, eyebrow and eyeliner pencils, and lipsticks can all be stored in the chilled compartment. This will extend the life of your polishes and make lip and eye pencils stiffer, resulting in sharper lines.

Oh my goodness! You have completed this guide. You can begin integrating them all in your life to achieve the flawless skin you've always desired. The knowledge you've gotten from this book will not only help you convert your skin into what you desire, but it will also help you save a lot of money by taking care of your skin at home. Good-luck!

Thank you for trusting me with your special kind of beauty!

Website: sheriseinc.me

YouTube: https://www.youtube.com/channel/UCM1efpATfpA4dHB97g4GPVQ

Instagram: https://www.instagram.com/She_rise_inc/

Facebook: https://www.facebook.com/sheriseinc.me/

Email: latoshatownsend@gmail.com